Deflame: A 30-Day Nutritional Blueprint to Combat Chronic Inflammation

Yakson Bobby

Table of Contents

Overview

Chronic inflammation is a silent epidemic, often lurking behind the scenes of various health issues, from arthritis and cardiovascular diseases to diabetes and even cancer. Unlike acute inflammation, which is a natural and necessary response to injury or infection, chronic inflammation persists over time, causing a continuous state of alert in the immune system. This prolonged inflammatory response can lead to tissue damage and exacerbate the progression of numerous diseases. It can manifest in subtle ways, such as persistent fatigue, digestive issues, or joint pain, making it easy to overlook until significant damage has occurred. The insidious nature of chronic inflammation means it can cause prolonged discomfort, lead to severe health complications, and significantly diminish one's quality of life.

In "Deflame: A 30-Day Nutritional Blueprint to Combat Chronic Inflammation," we embark on a transformative journey to reclaim your health through the power of nutrition. The book aims to shine a light on this hidden enemy and equip you with the knowledge and tools needed to combat it effectively. Our approach is rooted in science and practicality, providing a comprehensive understanding of how dietary choices influence inflammation and overall health. By addressing the root causes of inflammation, rather than merely treating its symptoms, we offer a sustainable path to improved well-being. This guide is designed for those who seek to not only alleviate the symptoms of chronic inflammation but also to prevent its recurrence, fostering long-term health and vitality.

The journey outlined in this book is not merely about a temporary diet change but aims to establish sustainable habits that will benefit you long-term. We recognize that quick fixes and fad diets often fail because they do not address the underlying issues or provide a realistic, maintainable lifestyle change. Instead, our plan focuses on integrating anti-inflammatory foods and practices into your daily routine, ensuring that the benefits extend far beyond the initial 30 days. By gradually adjusting your eating habits and making informed choices, you can create a lasting impact on your health, reducing inflammation and its associated risks.

Understanding the underlying causes of inflammation is crucial in learning how to counteract them through thoughtful dietary choices. Many common foods and lifestyle factors contribute to chronic inflammation, including processed foods, high sugar intake, and stress. By identifying and eliminating these triggers, and replacing them with nutrient-dense, anti-inflammatory foods, you can significantly reduce your inflammation levels. Our guide provides a clear, actionable plan to help you navigate this process, offering delicious recipes, meal plans, and practical tips to support your journey. With "Deflame: A 30-Day Nutritional Blueprint to Combat Chronic Inflammation," you can pave the way for a healthier, more vibrant life, free from the burdens of chronic inflammation.

Chapter 1: Understanding Inflammation

Inflammation is a fundamental biological response to injury, infection, or harmful stimuli. It is the body's natural defense mechanism designed to protect us and promote healing. When we get a cut, bruise, or infection, our immune system triggers an inflammatory response to eliminate the threat and repair the damaged tissue. This process involves an intricate interplay of cells and chemicals, orchestrated to localize and eradicate the invader, clear out dead cells, and initiate tissue repair. However, not all inflammation is beneficial. While acute inflammation is a necessary and short-term response, chronic inflammation can be detrimental to our health.

Chronic inflammation, unlike its acute counterpart, persists over a long period and can occur even when there is no apparent injury or infection. It is a slow, insidious process that can contribute to the development of various diseases, including arthritis, cardiovascular diseases, diabetes, and cancer. This type of inflammation often goes unnoticed until it has caused significant damage, leading to prolonged discomfort and severe health complications. Understanding the differences between acute and chronic inflammation, as well as the body's natural defense mechanisms, is crucial for recognizing when inflammation becomes harmful and how to address it effectively.

What is Inflammation?

Inflammation is the body's immediate response to injury or infection, aimed at protecting and healing the affected tissue. It is characterized by redness, heat, swelling, pain, and sometimes loss of function. These classic signs indicate that the immune system is actively working to contain and resolve the issue. Inflammation begins when immune cells release signaling molecules called cytokines, which attract other immune cells to the site of injury or infection. This cascade of events helps isolate the harmful agents, remove damaged cells, and initiate the healing process. Inflammation is an essential part of the body's defense, without which infections and injuries could become life-threatening.

There are two main types of inflammation: acute and chronic. Acute inflammation is short-term and usually resolves once the underlying cause is eliminated. It is a rapid response that occurs immediately after an injury or infection and lasts for a few hours to a few days. This type of inflammation is beneficial as it helps the body heal and recover quickly. Chronic inflammation, on the other hand, is long-term and can last for months or even years. It occurs when the immune system fails to eliminate the cause of inflammation or mistakenly targets healthy tissues. This persistent state of inflammation can lead to tissue damage and contribute to the development of chronic diseases.

Definition and Types: Acute vs. Chronic

Acute inflammation is a vital and immediate reaction to injury or infection, typically lasting a short period, from a few hours to a few days. This response is characterized by the familiar signs of inflammation: redness, heat, swelling, pain, and loss of function. These symptoms result from the increased blood flow and immune cell activity in the affected area, designed to eliminate pathogens, clear out damaged cells, and begin the healing process. For instance, when you cut your finger, the area becomes red and swollen as the immune system responds to prevent infection and promote repair. Acute inflammation is generally beneficial and resolves once the healing process is underway.

In contrast, chronic inflammation is a prolonged and often maladaptive response that can persist for months or even years. Unlike acute inflammation, which resolves once the initial threat is neutralized, chronic inflammation occurs when the immune system continues to respond as if there is a constant threat, even in the absence of an active infection or injury. This type of inflammation can arise from various factors, including ongoing exposure to irritants (such as smoking or pollution), chronic infections, autoimmune disorders, and prolonged stress. Chronic inflammation is less noticeable than acute inflammation but can cause ongoing damage to tissues and organs, contributing to diseases such as heart disease, diabetes, and cancer.

The Body's Natural Defense Mechanism

The body's natural defense mechanism, the immune system, is a complex network of cells, tissues, and organs that work together to protect us from harmful invaders. When the immune system detects an injury or infection, it triggers an inflammatory response to neutralize the threat and initiate healing. This response involves the release of various chemicals and the activation of immune cells, such as white blood cells, which work to eliminate the harmful agents and repair the damaged tissue. The inflammatory process is tightly regulated by the body to ensure that it is effective yet limited in scope and duration.

Inflammation is a crucial part of the immune response, but it must be carefully controlled to prevent excessive tissue damage. When the immune system functions correctly, inflammation resolves once the threat is neutralized, and the healing process begins. However, if the immune system is overactive or fails to regulate inflammation properly, it can lead to chronic inflammation. This prolonged inflammatory state can cause ongoing tissue damage and contribute to the development of various chronic diseases. Understanding how the body's natural defense mechanism works and the factors that influence inflammation is essential for maintaining optimal health and preventing chronic inflammation.

When Inflammation Becomes Harmful

Inflammation becomes harmful when it persists for an extended period or occurs inappropriately. Chronic inflammation can be triggered by various factors, including infections that the body cannot eliminate, ongoing exposure to harmful substances, autoimmune disorders, and lifestyle factors such as poor diet, lack of exercise, and chronic stress. Unlike acute inflammation, which is a beneficial and self-limiting response, chronic inflammation can lead to a continuous state of immune activation, causing tissue damage and contributing to the development of chronic diseases.

The harmful effects of chronic inflammation can manifest in different ways, depending on the tissues and organs involved. For example, in the case of cardiovascular diseases, chronic inflammation can lead to the buildup of plaques in the arteries, increasing the risk of heart attack and stroke. In diabetes, chronic inflammation can impair insulin signaling and contribute to insulin resistance. In autoimmune diseases, the immune system mistakenly targets healthy tissues, causing inflammation and damage. Recognizing the signs of chronic inflammation and understanding its underlying causes are crucial for taking proactive steps to reduce inflammation and protect overall health.

Causes and Triggers of Chronic Inflammation

Chronic inflammation is a complex condition influenced by various factors that can perpetuate the body's inflammatory response. Unlike acute inflammation, which serves a protective and healing purpose, chronic inflammation persists and can lead to a multitude of health issues. Understanding the root causes and triggers of chronic inflammation is crucial for developing effective strategies to combat it. These causes and triggers can be broadly categorized into dietary factors, lifestyle choices, environmental influences, and genetic predispositions. Each of these elements can contribute individually or synergistically to the maintenance and exacerbation of chronic inflammation.

Dietary Factors

The food we consume plays a significant role in either promoting or mitigating inflammation. Diets high in processed foods, refined sugars, and unhealthy fats, such as trans fats and saturated fats, can trigger and sustain inflammatory responses in the body. Processed foods often contain additives, preservatives, and artificial ingredients that can irritate the digestive system and disrupt the balance of gut microbiota, leading to inflammation. On the other hand, a diet rich in anti-inflammatory foods, such as fruits, vegetables, whole grains, lean proteins, and healthy fats like omega-3 fatty acids, can help reduce inflammation. Nutrient-dense foods provide essential vitamins, minerals, and antioxidants that support the immune system and help regulate inflammatory processes.

Lifestyle Choices

Lifestyle choices significantly impact the body's inflammatory response. Physical inactivity, for instance, can lead to weight gain and obesity, which are closely linked to chronic inflammation. Excess body fat, especially visceral fat, produces inflammatory molecules called adipokines that contribute to systemic inflammation. Conversely, regular physical activity helps reduce inflammation by promoting weight loss, improving circulation, and enhancing the body's anti-inflammatory responses. Additionally, chronic stress is a major contributor to inflammation. Stress triggers the release of cortisol and other stress hormones, which, when elevated for prolonged periods, can lead to persistent inflammation. Managing stress through techniques such as mindfulness, meditation, and regular exercise is crucial for reducing inflammation.

Environmental Influences

The environment we live in can also influence the levels of inflammation in our bodies. Exposure to pollutants, chemicals, and toxins can provoke inflammatory responses. Air pollution, for example, contains particulate matter and other pollutants that, when inhaled, can cause respiratory inflammation and systemic inflammatory effects. Similarly, exposure to industrial chemicals, pesticides, and heavy metals can disrupt normal cellular function and lead to chronic inflammation. In addition, a sedentary lifestyle often associated with urban living can exacerbate these effects. Reducing exposure to environmental toxins and maintaining a clean living space can help mitigate inflammation.

Genetic Predisposition

Genetic factors can predispose individuals to chronic inflammation and influence how the body responds to inflammatory triggers. Certain genetic variations can affect the immune system's ability to regulate inflammation, making some people more susceptible to chronic inflammatory conditions. For instance, genetic predispositions can influence the production and activity of cytokines, proteins that play a key role in the inflammatory response. Additionally, hereditary conditions such as autoimmune diseases, where the immune system mistakenly attacks healthy tissues, can lead to chronic inflammation. While genetic predisposition cannot be changed, understanding one's genetic risks can help tailor lifestyle and dietary interventions to manage and reduce inflammation more effectively.

Chronic inflammation is a multifaceted condition influenced by diet, lifestyle choices, environmental factors, and genetic predispositions. By identifying and addressing these causes and triggers, individuals can take proactive steps to reduce inflammation and improve their overall health.

Health Implications of Chronic Inflammation

Chronic inflammation is a persistent and often subtle condition that can have profound effects on health. Unlike acute inflammation, which is a short-term and necessary response to injury or infection, chronic inflammation is a slow and prolonged state that can cause significant damage to the body over time. The implications of chronic inflammation are far-reaching, affecting various systems and leading to a host of diseases and health complications. Understanding these implications is crucial for recognizing the importance of managing and reducing chronic inflammation.

Links to Common Diseases

Chronic inflammation has been linked to a wide range of common diseases, many of which are serious and life-threatening. Cardiovascular diseases, including heart disease and stroke, are strongly associated with chronic inflammation. Inflammatory processes contribute to the development and progression of atherosclerosis, where plaque builds up in the arteries, leading to blockages that can result in heart attacks or strokes. Similarly, chronic inflammation plays a critical role in the onset of type 2 diabetes by interfering with insulin signaling and contributing to insulin resistance. Cancer is another major disease linked to chronic inflammation. Inflammatory cells can produce chemicals that promote tumor growth and metastasis. Furthermore, autoimmune diseases like rheumatoid arthritis and lupus involve chronic inflammation as the immune system mistakenly attacks healthy tissues. Understanding the connection between chronic inflammation and these diseases highlights the importance of addressing inflammation to prevent and manage these conditions.

Symptoms and Signs to Watch For

Chronic inflammation can be insidious, often presenting with subtle and varied symptoms that can be easily overlooked or mistaken for other conditions. Common signs of chronic inflammation include persistent fatigue, unexplained aches and pains, and digestive issues such as bloating, diarrhea, or constipation. Individuals may also experience frequent infections or illnesses, as chronic inflammation can weaken the immune system's ability to fight off pathogens. Other symptoms include skin problems like rashes or acne, mood disorders such as depression and anxiety, and weight gain, particularly around the abdomen. Recognizing these symptoms and seeking medical advice can help in early detection and management of chronic inflammation. It is important to note that these symptoms can vary widely among individuals, and chronic inflammation may manifest differently depending on the underlying cause and the body's response.

Long-Term Effects on Overall Health

The long-term effects of chronic inflammation on overall health can be devastating, contributing to a decline in quality of life and increased risk of mortality. Chronic inflammation can lead to continuous tissue damage and dysfunction in various organs, including the heart, brain, liver, and kidneys. Over time, this can result in the loss of function and the development of chronic diseases that significantly impair daily activities and overall well-being. For example, chronic inflammation in the arteries can lead to atherosclerosis, increasing the risk of heart attacks and strokes. In the brain, chronic inflammation is associated with neurodegenerative diseases such as Alzheimer's disease and Parkinson's disease, leading to cognitive decline and loss of motor function. In the liver, chronic inflammation can cause fatty liver disease and cirrhosis, while in the kidneys, it can lead to chronic kidney disease and eventual kidney failure. Additionally, chronic inflammation can accelerate the aging process and contribute to the development of age-related diseases. Addressing chronic inflammation through lifestyle changes, dietary adjustments, and medical interventions is crucial for maintaining long-term health and preventing these adverse outcomes.

Chronic inflammation is a pervasive and harmful condition that can lead to a wide range of serious health problems. By understanding its links to common diseases, recognizing the symptoms and signs, and acknowledging its long-term effects on overall health, individuals can take proactive steps to manage and reduce chronic inflammation, thereby improving their quality of life and longevity.

Chapter 2: The Science Behind the Anti-Inflammatory Diet

The relationship between diet and inflammation is a complex and fascinating area of nutritional science. What we eat profoundly affects our body's inflammatory processes, with certain foods and nutrients capable of either promoting or reducing inflammation. The study of nutritional biochemistry provides insights into how different nutrients interact with our body's systems, influencing health and disease outcomes. By understanding these interactions, we can make informed dietary choices that help manage and reduce chronic inflammation, ultimately improving overall health and preventing disease.

The anti-inflammatory diet is not just a temporary eating plan but a sustainable approach to long-term health. It involves consuming a variety of foods that provide essential nutrients, antioxidants, and phytochemicals that work synergistically to combat inflammation. This chapter delves into the science behind these dietary components, exploring how specific nutrients function at the biochemical level to reduce inflammation. We will also examine the critical role of antioxidants and phytochemicals, as well as the impact of gut health and the microbiome on inflammation, to provide a comprehensive understanding of how diet can be a powerful tool in managing chronic inflammation.

Nutritional Biochemistry

Nutritional biochemistry explores the intricate relationship between the nutrients we consume and our body's biochemical processes, particularly in how they influence inflammation. Certain nutrients, such as omega-3 fatty acids, vitamin D, magnesium, and polyphenols, possess potent anti-inflammatory properties that help regulate and reduce chronic inflammation. These nutrients work by modulating the immune response, inhibiting the production of pro-inflammatory molecules, and promoting anti-inflammatory pathways. Additionally, antioxidants and phytochemicals, naturally occurring compounds in plants, protect cells from oxidative damage and further reduce inflammation.

Understanding these interactions allows us to make informed dietary choices that support our health, reduce the risk of inflammation-related diseases, and enhance overall well-being.

Anti-inflammatory Nutrients and Their Mechanisms

Nutritional biochemistry reveals that certain nutrients have powerful anti-inflammatory properties, which can help mitigate the chronic inflammation that underlies many diseases. Omega-3 fatty acids, found in fatty fish, flaxseeds, and walnuts, are among the most potent anti-inflammatory nutrients. They work by inhibiting the production of inflammatory molecules such as prostaglandins and leukotrienes. Omega-3s also promote the production of anti-inflammatory molecules, helping to balance the body's inflammatory response. Regular consumption of omega-3-rich foods has been shown to reduce inflammation markers in the body, benefiting conditions such as heart disease, arthritis, and inflammatory bowel disease.

In addition to omega-3 fatty acids, other nutrients such as vitamin D, magnesium, and polyphenols play crucial roles in reducing inflammation. Vitamin D, obtained from sunlight and certain foods like fatty fish and fortified dairy products, modulates the immune system and reduces the production of pro-inflammatory cytokines. Magnesium, found in leafy greens, nuts, and seeds, helps regulate inflammation by balancing the body's calcium levels and supporting proper muscle and nerve function. Polyphenols, abundant in fruits, vegetables, tea, and red wine, have antioxidant properties that protect cells from damage and reduce inflammation by inhibiting inflammatory pathways. Together, these nutrients form a powerful arsenal against chronic inflammation.

Role of Antioxidants and Phytochemicals

Antioxidants are compounds that protect the body from oxidative stress, a condition where an excess of free radicals causes cellular damage and inflammation. Free radicals are unstable molecules that can damage cells, proteins, and DNA, contributing to the development of chronic diseases. Antioxidants neutralize free radicals, preventing them from causing harm. Vitamin C, vitamin E, and selenium are well-known antioxidants that help reduce inflammation. Vitamin C, found in citrus fruits, berries, and leafy greens, enhances the immune system and aids in the repair of damaged tissues. Vitamin E, present in nuts, seeds, and vegetable oils, protects cell membranes from oxidative damage. Selenium, found in Brazil nuts, seafood, and eggs, supports the production of antioxidant enzymes.

Phytochemicals, naturally occurring compounds found in plants, also play a significant role in combating inflammation. These compounds include flavonoids, carotenoids, and glucosinolates, each with unique anti-inflammatory properties. Flavonoids, found in fruits, vegetables, tea, and dark chocolate, have been shown to reduce inflammation by inhibiting enzymes involved in the inflammatory process. Carotenoids, present in colorful fruits and vegetables like carrots, sweet potatoes, and spinach, protect cells from oxidative damage and reduce inflammation. Glucosinolates, found in cruciferous vegetables like broccoli, cabbage, and kale, support detoxification processes in the body and reduce inflammation. Incorporating a variety of antioxidant-rich and phytochemical-rich foods into the diet is essential for managing chronic inflammation.

Gut Health and the Microbiome's Impact on Inflammation

The gut microbiome, the diverse community of microorganisms residing in the digestive tract, plays a critical role in regulating inflammation. A healthy and balanced gut microbiome supports the immune system, helps digest food, and protects against harmful pathogens. However, an imbalance in the gut microbiome, known as dysbiosis, can contribute to chronic inflammation. Factors such as poor diet, antibiotic use, and stress can disrupt the balance of gut bacteria, leading to increased intestinal permeability, often referred to as "leaky gut." This condition allows harmful substances to enter the bloodstream, triggering an immune response and promoting inflammation.

Maintaining a healthy gut microbiome is essential for reducing inflammation and promoting overall health. Consuming probiotic-rich foods, such as yogurt, kefir, sauerkraut, and kimchi, can help replenish beneficial bacteria in the gut. Probiotics are live microorganisms that provide health benefits when consumed in adequate amounts. They help restore the balance of the gut microbiome, enhance the intestinal barrier function, and reduce inflammation. Prebiotics, found in foods like garlic, onions, bananas, and asparagus, are non-digestible fibers that serve as food for beneficial gut bacteria. By promoting the growth of these bacteria, prebiotics support a healthy gut environment and reduce inflammation.

The science behind the anti-inflammatory diet emphasizes the importance of specific nutrients, antioxidants, phytochemicals, and gut health in managing chronic inflammation. By understanding the biochemical mechanisms of these dietary components, individuals can make informed choices that support their health and reduce the risk of inflammation-related diseases. The anti-inflammatory diet is a sustainable approach to long-term health, providing a foundation for a vibrant and disease-free life.

Foods that Fuel Inflammation

The foods we eat can significantly impact our body's inflammatory response. While some foods possess anti-inflammatory properties, others can exacerbate inflammation, contributing to chronic health issues. The typical Western diet, characterized by high consumption of processed foods, sugars, and unhealthy fats, has been closely linked to increased levels of inflammation. These dietary habits can disrupt the body's balance, leading to a persistent inflammatory state that underlies many chronic diseases. Understanding which foods fuel inflammation is crucial for making healthier dietary choices that promote overall well-being and reduce the risk of inflammation-related health problems.

In this section, we will explore specific categories of foods that are known to contribute to inflammation. Processed foods and trans fats, sugars and refined carbohydrates, and common allergens and sensitivities are all significant culprits. By examining how these foods affect our body, we can gain a clearer understanding of the importance of dietary modifications in managing and preventing chronic inflammation. Awareness of these inflammatory triggers empowers individuals to make informed decisions about their diet, fostering a healthier, more balanced lifestyle.

Processed Foods and Trans Fats

Processed foods, which include a wide range of packaged and prepared foods, are often laden with unhealthy ingredients that fuel inflammation. These foods typically contain high levels of trans fats, artificial additives, preservatives, and other inflammatory agents. Trans fats, in particular, are known to increase levels of low-density lipoprotein (LDL) cholesterol, commonly referred to as "bad" cholesterol, while lowering high-density lipoprotein (HDL) cholesterol, or "good" cholesterol. This imbalance can lead to the buildup of arterial plaque, promoting heart disease and chronic inflammation. Moreover, processed foods often lack essential nutrients and fiber, further contributing to poor health outcomes and sustained inflammation.

Sugars and Refined Carbohydrates

Sugars and refined carbohydrates are major contributors to chronic inflammation. These substances are rapidly absorbed into the bloodstream, causing spikes in blood sugar levels and subsequent insulin release. Over time, high intake of sugars and refined carbs can lead to insulin resistance, a condition where the body's cells become less responsive to insulin. This resistance is a key driver of inflammation and is associated with the development of type 2 diabetes, obesity, and metabolic syndrome. Foods high in refined sugars, such as sugary beverages, pastries, and white bread, also contribute to oxidative stress and the production of advanced glycation end products (AGEs), which further exacerbate inflammation and damage tissues.

Common Allergens and Sensitivities

Common allergens and food sensitivities can also play a significant role in fueling inflammation. Foods such as gluten, dairy, soy, and certain nuts can trigger inflammatory responses in individuals who are sensitive or allergic to them. When these allergens are consumed, the immune system may mistakenly identify them as harmful invaders, leading to an inflammatory response. This reaction can cause a range of symptoms, from digestive issues and skin rashes to joint pain and fatigue. Chronic exposure to food allergens can lead to sustained inflammation and contribute to the development of chronic inflammatory conditions, such as irritable bowel syndrome (IBS) and autoimmune diseases. Identifying and eliminating these trigger foods from the diet can help reduce inflammation and improve overall health.

Foods that Fight Inflammation

In contrast to foods that fuel inflammation, certain foods possess powerful anti-inflammatory properties that can help manage and reduce chronic inflammation.

Incorporating these foods into your diet can enhance your overall health, prevent the onset of inflammatory diseases, and improve your body's ability to combat inflammation naturally. These beneficial foods are rich in essential nutrients, antioxidants, and bioactive compounds that support the immune system and promote a balanced inflammatory response. Understanding and incorporating these foods into your daily meals can be a proactive step towards achieving optimal health and well-being.

In this section, we will explore three key categories of anti-inflammatory foods: fruits and vegetables, omega-3 fatty acids, and herbs and spices. Each of these categories offers unique compounds and benefits that work synergistically to reduce inflammation and protect against chronic diseases. By emphasizing these foods in your diet, you can harness their natural anti-inflammatory properties and support your body's health at a cellular level.

Fruits and Vegetables

Fruits and vegetables are among the most potent anti-inflammatory foods due to their high content of vitamins, minerals, fiber, and phytochemicals. These nutrients play a crucial role in reducing inflammation and supporting overall health. For example, leafy greens like spinach and kale are rich in antioxidants such as vitamin C, vitamin E, and beta-carotene, which neutralize free radicals and reduce oxidative stress. Berries, including blueberries, strawberries, and raspberries, contain anthocyanins and other polyphenols that have been shown to lower inflammatory markers in the body. Additionally, cruciferous vegetables like broccoli, Brussels sprouts, and cauliflower provide sulforaphane, a compound that helps modulate the body's inflammatory response and supports detoxification processes.

Omega-3 Fatty Acids

Omega-3 fatty acids, primarily found in fatty fish like salmon, mackerel, and sardines, as well as in flaxseeds, chia seeds, and walnuts, are essential fats with strong anti-inflammatory effects. These fatty acids, particularly eicosapentaenoic acid (EPA) and docosahexaenoic acid (DHA), play a crucial role in reducing the production of inflammatory molecules such as prostaglandins and leukotrienes. Omega-3s also promote the synthesis of anti-inflammatory molecules called resolvins and proteins, which help resolve inflammation and support the healing process. Regular consumption of omega-3-rich foods has been associated with lower levels of inflammation and reduced risk of chronic diseases such as heart disease, arthritis, and inflammatory bowel disease. Incorporating these healthy fats into your diet can help balance the body's inflammatory response and improve overall health.

Herbs and Spices with Anti-Inflammatory Properties

Herbs and spices are not only flavor enhancers but also powerful anti-inflammatory agents. Many herbs and spices contain bioactive compounds that can significantly reduce inflammation and support health. Turmeric, for example, contains curcumin, a compound with potent anti-inflammatory and antioxidant properties. Curcumin inhibits several inflammatory pathways in the body, making it effective in managing conditions such as arthritis, metabolic syndrome, and even certain cancers. Ginger, another widely used spice, contains gingerol, which has been shown to reduce inflammation and oxidative stress. It can help alleviate symptoms of inflammatory conditions like osteoarthritis and irritable bowel syndrome.

Other herbs and spices with notable anti-inflammatory properties include garlic, which contains sulfur compounds that modulate the immune response and reduce inflammation, and cinnamon, which has antioxidant properties that help reduce inflammation and protect against cellular damage. Incorporating a variety of these herbs and spices into your daily meals can enhance the anti-inflammatory benefits of your diet, making it more effective in preventing and managing chronic inflammation.

Chapter 3: Crafting Your 30-Day Blueprint

Creating a sustainable and effective anti-inflammatory diet involves more than just choosing the right foods; it requires a well-thought-out plan that aligns with your lifestyle and health goals. Crafting a 30-day blueprint is about setting realistic, achievable objectives and creating an environment that supports your journey towards better health. This chapter will guide you through the essential steps of assessing your current diet and lifestyle, defining clear and attainable objectives, and establishing a supportive environment that fosters long-term success. By following these steps, you can lay a strong foundation for a transformative dietary shift that not only reduces inflammation but also enhances your overall well-being.

Setting Realistic Goals

Setting realistic goals is the cornerstone of any successful health transformation. Unrealistic expectations can lead to frustration and abandonment of the plan, while achievable goals can keep you motivated and on track. To set realistic goals, it's essential to start by understanding where you currently stand in terms of your diet and lifestyle.

Assessing Your Current Diet and Lifestyle

The first step in crafting your 30-day blueprint is to take a comprehensive look at your current dietary habits and lifestyle. Begin by keeping a food diary for a week, recording everything you eat and drink, as well as your meal times and portion sizes. This record will help you identify patterns and pinpoint areas that need improvement. Pay attention to the types of foods you consume, the frequency of processed and sugary foods, and the balance of macronutrients in your meals. Additionally, consider your lifestyle factors such as physical activity levels, sleep patterns, and stress management practices. Understanding these elements will provide a clear picture of where you are starting from and highlight the specific changes needed to reduce inflammation and improve health.

Defining Your Objectives

Once you have a clear understanding of your current diet and lifestyle, the next step is to define your objectives. Your goals should be specific, measurable, achievable, relevant, and time-bound (SMART). Start by identifying the primary reasons you want to adopt an anti-inflammatory diet. Are you looking to reduce symptoms of a chronic condition, lose weight, increase energy levels, or improve overall health? Be specific about what you want to achieve and set measurable targets. For example, instead of setting a vague goal like "eat healthier," aim for "increase vegetable intake to five servings per day" or "reduce sugar consumption by half." Make sure your goals are realistic and attainable within the 30-day timeframe. Setting small, incremental goals will help you build momentum and stay motivated throughout the process.

Creating a Supportive Environment

A supportive environment is crucial for the success of your 30-day blueprint. This involves not only creating a physical space that facilitates healthy eating but also seeking emotional and social support. Start by organizing your kitchen and pantry to remove inflammatory foods and stock up on anti-inflammatory options. Clear out processed foods, sugary snacks, and trans fats, and replace them with fresh fruits, vegetables, whole grains, lean proteins, and healthy fats. Invest in quality kitchen tools and gadgets that make meal preparation easier and more enjoyable.

In addition to creating a conducive physical environment, seek support from family, friends, and community resources. Share your goals with your loved ones and ask for their encouragement and understanding. Consider joining a support group or online community focused on anti-inflammatory diets and healthy living. These groups can provide valuable advice, motivation, and a sense of accountability. Surrounding yourself with positive influences and resources will help you stay committed to your goals and navigate any challenges that arise during your 30-day journey.

Setting realistic goals is a multi-step process that begins with assessing your current diet and lifestyle, defining clear and achievable objectives, and creating a supportive environment. By following these steps, you can establish a strong foundation for your anti-inflammatory diet and set yourself up for long-term success. The next sections of this chapter will delve deeper into meal planning, preparation, and tips to help you stay on track throughout your 30-day journey.

Meal Planning and Preparation

Effective meal planning and preparation are critical components of a successful anti-inflammatory diet. By organizing your meals in advance, you can ensure that you have healthy, anti-inflammatory foods readily available, making it easier to adhere to your dietary goals. This section will guide you through the process of creating weekly meal plans, compiling comprehensive shopping lists, stocking your pantry with essential items, and implementing time-saving tips to accommodate busy schedules. With careful planning and preparation, you can make healthy eating an effortless and enjoyable part of your daily routine.

Weekly Meal Plans

Creating a weekly meal plan is the first step towards consistent and balanced eating. Start by selecting a variety of anti-inflammatory foods to include in your meals. Aim to incorporate a wide range of fruits, vegetables, whole grains, lean proteins, and healthy fats to ensure you receive a broad spectrum of nutrients. Plan your meals around these foods, considering breakfast, lunch, dinner, and snacks.

Begin by outlining a basic framework for the week. For instance, you might decide to have oatmeal with berries and nuts for breakfast, a salad with lean protein for lunch, and a vegetable-rich stir-fry for dinner. Incorporate different themes or cuisines to keep your meals interesting and diverse. For example, you could have Mediterranean Mondays, Taco Tuesdays, and Stir-Fry Fridays. By establishing a routine, you can streamline your planning process and ensure you have all the necessary ingredients on hand.

Shopping Lists and Pantry Essentials

Once you have your weekly meal plan, the next step is to create a detailed shopping list. A well-organized shopping list not only saves time but also ensures that you don't forget any essential items. Divide your list into categories such as produce, dairy, proteins, grains, and pantry staples. This categorization makes shopping more efficient and helps you quickly locate items in the store.

Stocking your pantry with anti-inflammatory essentials is crucial for quick and easy meal preparation. Keep a variety of whole grains such as quinoa, brown rice, and oats, as well as canned beans and legumes like chickpeas and lentils. Healthy fats like olive oil, avocado oil, and nuts should also be pantry staples. Additionally, stock up on herbs and spices known for their anti-inflammatory properties, such as turmeric, ginger, garlic, and cinnamon. Having these essentials on hand allows you to whip up healthy meals without needing to run to the store frequently.

Time-Saving Tips for Busy Schedules

For many people, finding time to prepare healthy meals can be challenging, especially with a busy schedule. However, with some strategic planning and time-saving techniques, you can ensure that healthy eating fits seamlessly into your routine. One effective strategy is batch cooking. Set aside a few hours each week to prepare large quantities of food that can be stored and eaten throughout the week. Cook grains, proteins, and vegetables in bulk, and portion them into individual containers for quick grab-and-go meals.

Another useful tip is to prep ingredients ahead of time. Wash, chop, and store vegetables as soon as you bring them home from the store. This reduces the time needed to prepare meals during the week. Additionally, consider investing in kitchen gadgets that can save time, such as a slow cooker, instant pot, or food processor. These tools can simplify meal preparation and cooking, allowing you to prepare healthy meals with minimal effort.

Finally, make use of leftovers creatively. Instead of seeing leftovers as repetitive, view them as building blocks for new meals. Leftover roasted vegetables can be added to salads, grain bowls, or omelets. Cooked chicken can be transformed into tacos, sandwiches, or soups. By repurposing leftovers, you can reduce food waste and save time on meal preparation.

Effective meal planning and preparation are essential for maintaining a consistent anti-inflammatory diet. By creating weekly meal plans, organizing comprehensive shopping lists, stocking your pantry with essentials, and implementing time-saving techniques, you can make healthy eating a manageable and enjoyable part of your busy lifestyle. The following sections will provide detailed recipes and further tips to help you stay on track and achieve your health goals.

Chapter 4: Week 1 – Detox and Reset

Embarking on an anti-inflammatory diet begins with a week dedicated to detoxing and resetting your body. This initial phase is crucial for eliminating harmful substances and laying the foundation for healthier eating habits. By focusing on whole foods, you can nourish your body with essential nutrients, reduce inflammation, and start feeling more energized and revitalized. This week sets the stage for the rest of the journey, ensuring that you begin on the right foot with a clean slate. The key components of this week include eliminating processed foods, incorporating fresh produce, and understanding the importance of hydration.

Focus on Whole Foods

Whole foods are the cornerstone of a healthy, anti-inflammatory diet. Unlike processed foods, which are often stripped of their nutrients and filled with additives, whole foods are nutrient-dense and minimally processed. They provide the vitamins, minerals, antioxidants, and fiber your body needs to function optimally and combat inflammation. By focusing on whole foods, you can ensure that you are nourishing your body with the best possible fuel, supporting your overall health and well-being.

Eliminating Processed Foods

The first step in detoxing and resetting your diet is to eliminate processed foods. Processed foods are typically high in unhealthy fats, sugars, sodium, and artificial ingredients, all of which can contribute to inflammation. These foods often contain trans fats, which increase levels of bad cholesterol and promote inflammation, as well as refined sugars and carbohydrates that cause spikes in blood sugar and insulin levels. Additionally, many processed foods contain preservatives, colorings, and flavorings that can disrupt your body's natural processes and exacerbate inflammation.

To eliminate processed foods, start by reading food labels and avoiding products with long lists of ingredients, especially those with names you cannot pronounce. Focus on whole, natural foods that are as close to their original state as possible. This means choosing fresh fruits and vegetables, whole grains, lean proteins, and healthy fats over packaged snacks, ready meals, and sugary treats. Cleaning out your pantry and refrigerator of processed foods and replacing them with whole food alternatives can help you make healthier choices more easily.

Incorporating Fresh Produce

Fresh produce is a vital part of an anti-inflammatory diet, offering a wide array of nutrients that help reduce inflammation and support overall health. Fruits and vegetables are rich in vitamins, minerals, fiber, and antioxidants, all of which play a role in combating inflammation. For example, leafy greens like spinach and kale are high in antioxidants such as vitamin C and beta-carotene, which help neutralize free radicals and reduce oxidative stress. Berries, such as blueberries and strawberries, are packed with polyphenols that have been shown to lower inflammation markers in the body.

Incorporating a variety of colorful fruits and vegetables into your meals ensures that you receive a broad spectrum of nutrients. Aim to fill half your plate with produce at each meal, and try to include at least one serving of fruits or vegetables in every snack. Experiment with different types of produce to keep your meals interesting and diverse. Fresh produce can be enjoyed in numerous ways, from salads and smoothies to roasted vegetables and fruit parfaits. By making fruits and vegetables a central part of your diet, you can enhance your intake of anti-inflammatory nutrients and support your body's natural detoxification processes.

Hydration and Its Importance

Hydration is an often-overlooked aspect of an anti-inflammatory diet, but it is crucial for maintaining optimal health and supporting detoxification. Water plays a vital role in every cell and system in the body, including the regulation of inflammation. Staying adequately hydrated helps flush out toxins, transport nutrients, and maintain the health of your joints and tissues. Dehydration, on the other hand, can exacerbate inflammation and impair your body's ability to function properly.

To ensure you are properly hydrated, aim to drink at least eight glasses of water per day, or more if you are physically active or live in a hot climate. Herbal teas and water-rich foods like cucumbers, watermelon, and oranges can also contribute to your daily hydration needs. Avoid sugary drinks and excessive caffeine, as these can dehydrate the body and promote inflammation. Starting your day with a glass of water and drinking regularly throughout the day can help you maintain consistent hydration levels. Keeping a reusable water bottle with you can serve as a reminder to drink more water and make it easier to stay hydrated.

The first week of your anti-inflammatory diet is dedicated to detoxing and resetting your body by focusing on whole foods. By eliminating processed foods, incorporating fresh produce, and prioritizing hydration, you can reduce inflammation, enhance your health, and set the stage for a successful dietary transformation. The following sections will provide specific meal plans, recipes, and tips to help you navigate this initial phase and continue your journey towards better health.

Simple, Nourishing Recipes

Embarking on an anti-inflammatory diet requires a collection of simple yet nourishing recipes that you can easily incorporate into your daily routine. The goal is to enjoy delicious meals that are quick to prepare and packed with anti-inflammatory ingredients. This section provides a variety of recipes for breakfast, lunch, dinner, and snacks, along with smoothies and detox drinks, to help you navigate the first week of your new eating plan. These recipes are designed to be straightforward and enjoyable, ensuring that you can maintain your dietary changes without feeling overwhelmed.

Breakfast, Lunch, Dinner, and Snacks

Breakfast

Starting your day with a nutrient-rich breakfast sets the tone for healthy eating throughout the day. Here are a few easy breakfast options:

1. Overnight Oats with Berries and Nuts

- **Ingredients**: Rolled oats, almond milk, chia seeds, fresh berries, chopped nuts, honey (optional).
- **Preparation**: Combine oats, almond milk, and chia seeds in a jar. Refrigerate overnight. In the morning, top with fresh berries and nuts. Drizzle with honey if desired.

2. Spinach and Avocado Smoothie

- **Ingredients**: Fresh spinach, ripe avocado, banana, almond milk, a scoop of protein powder (optional).
- **Preparation**: Blend all ingredients until smooth. Enjoy immediately.

Lunch

A balanced lunch that includes lean protein, healthy fats, and plenty of vegetables will keep you energized and satisfied.

1. Quinoa and Black Bean Salad

- **Ingredients**: Cooked quinoa, black beans, cherry tomatoes, cucumber, red bell pepper, red onion, fresh cilantro, olive oil, lime juice, salt, and pepper.
- **Preparation**: Combine all ingredients in a large bowl. Toss with olive oil and lime juice. Season with salt and pepper to taste.

2. Turkey and Avocado Wrap

- **Ingredients**: Whole grain wrap, sliced turkey breast, avocado, mixed greens, sliced tomato, hummus.
- **Preparation**: Spread hummus on the wrap. Layer with turkey, avocado, greens, and tomato. Roll up tightly and slice in half.

Dinner

For dinner, focus on hearty yet healthy dishes that incorporate plenty of vegetables and lean proteins.

1. Baked Salmon with Roasted Vegetables

- **Ingredients**: Salmon filets, olive oil, lemon juice, garlic, fresh herbs (such as dill or parsley), mixed vegetables (such as broccoli, carrots, and bell peppers).

- **Preparation**: Preheat oven to 400°F (200°C). Place salmon on a baking sheet, drizzle with olive oil and lemon juice, and sprinkle with garlic and herbs. Arrange vegetables around the salmon, drizzle with olive oil, and season with salt and pepper. Bake for 20-25 minutes until salmon is cooked through and vegetables are tender.

2. Stir-Fried Tofu with Vegetables

- **Ingredients**: Firm tofu, mixed vegetables (such as bell peppers, snap peas, and carrots), soy sauce or tamari, sesame oil, garlic, ginger, cooked brown rice.

- **Preparation**: Press and cube tofu. In a hot pan, sauté garlic and ginger in sesame oil. Add tofu and cook until browned. Add vegetables and soy sauce, stir-frying until vegetables are tender-crisp. Serve over brown rice.

Snacks

Healthy snacks help keep your energy levels stable between meals.

1. Apple Slices with Almond Butter

- **Ingredients**: Apple slices, almond butter.
- **Preparation**: Slice an apple and serve with a side of almond butter for dipping.

2. Greek Yogurt with Honey and Walnuts

- **Ingredients**: Plain Greek yogurt, honey, chopped walnuts.

- **Preparation**: Top a bowl of Greek yogurt with a drizzle of honey and a sprinkle of chopped walnuts.

Smoothies and Detox Drinks

Smoothies and detox drinks are excellent for incorporating a variety of fruits and vegetables into your diet. They are quick to prepare and perfect for a nutrient boost.

1. Green Detox Smoothie

- **Ingredients**: Kale, cucumber, green apple, lemon juice, ginger, coconut water.
- **Preparation**: Blend all ingredients until smooth. Drink immediately for the best nutritional benefits.

2. Beet and Berry Smoothie

- **Ingredients**: Cooked beetroot, mixed berries (such as blueberries, raspberries, and strawberries), banana, almond milk, chia seeds.

- **Preparation**: Blend all ingredients until smooth. Serve chilled.

3. Turmeric Ginger Tea

- **Ingredients**: Fresh turmeric root, fresh ginger root, lemon juice, honey, hot water.
- **Preparation**: Slice turmeric and ginger root thinly. Add to a pot of hot water and simmer for 10 minutes. Strain into a cup, add lemon juice and honey to taste.

Easy-to-Make Dishes for the First Week

Starting with easy-to-make dishes ensures you can quickly adapt to your new diet without spending too much time in the kitchen.

1. Chickpea and Spinach Stew

- **Ingredients**: Canned chickpeas, fresh spinach, onion, garlic, tomatoes, vegetable broth, olive oil, cumin, paprika, salt, and pepper.

- **Preparation**: Sauté onion and garlic in olive oil until softened. Add chickpeas, tomatoes, and vegetable broth. Season with cumin, paprika, salt, and pepper. Simmer for 15-20 minutes. Stir in spinach and cook until wilted. Serve hot.

2. Lentil Soup

- **Ingredients**: Lentils, carrots, celery, onion, garlic, vegetable broth, bay leaf, thyme, olive oil, salt, and pepper.
- **Preparation**: Sauté onion, garlic, carrots, and celery in olive oil until softened. Add lentils, vegetable broth, bay leaf, and thyme. Season with salt and pepper. Simmer until lentils are tender, about 30 minutes. Remove bay leaf before serving.

3. Stuffed Bell Peppers

- **Ingredients**: Bell peppers, quinoa, black beans, corn, tomatoes, onion, garlic, cumin, chili powder, shredded cheese (optional).

- **Preparation**: Preheat oven to 375°F (190°C). Cut the tops off the bell peppers and remove seeds. Sauté onion and garlic in olive oil, then add quinoa, black beans, corn, tomatoes, cumin, and chili powder. Stuff peppers with the mixture and place in a baking dish. Top with shredded cheese if desired. Bake for 25-30 minutes until peppers are tender.

By incorporating these simple, nourishing recipes into your first week, you can ensure a smooth transition into your anti-inflammatory diet. These meals are designed to be easy to prepare, delicious, and packed with nutrients that will help reduce inflammation and improve your overall health.

Chapter 5: Week 2 – Building Anti-Inflammatory Habits

As you transition into the second week of your anti-inflammatory journey, the focus shifts to building long-lasting habits that will continue to support your health. This week is about solidifying the foundation you laid in Week 1 by introducing powerful anti-inflammatory superfoods, creating recipes that highlight these ingredients, and understanding how to balance macronutrients for optimal health. By the end of this week, you will have a robust toolkit of foods and practices that can help keep inflammation at bay and promote overall well-being.

Introducing Anti-Inflammatory Superfoods

Anti-inflammatory superfoods are nutrient-dense ingredients that have been shown to reduce inflammation and support overall health. Incorporating these superfoods into your diet can enhance your body's ability to fight inflammation and improve various health markers. Here are some key superfoods to add to your diet:

Turmeric

- Known for its active compound curcumin, turmeric has potent anti-inflammatory and antioxidant properties. It can help reduce symptoms of arthritis, digestive disorders, and other inflammatory conditions. Incorporate turmeric into your meals by adding it to soups, stews, and smoothies, or by making a warming turmeric tea.

Blueberries

- Blueberries are rich in antioxidants, particularly anthocyanins, which help reduce oxidative stress and inflammation. These berries are also high in fiber and vitamin C, making them a great addition to your diet. Enjoy blueberries as a snack, in smoothies, or mixed into yogurt or oatmeal.

Salmon

- Salmon is an excellent source of omega-3 fatty acids, which are essential for reducing inflammation. These healthy fats help lower the risk of chronic diseases such as heart disease and arthritis. Include salmon in your diet by grilling, baking, or pan-searing it, and pair it with a variety of vegetables for a balanced meal.

Leafy Greens

- Leafy greens like spinach, kale, and Swiss chard are loaded with vitamins, minerals, and antioxidants that support overall health and reduce inflammation. These greens are versatile and can be used in salads, smoothies, and cooked dishes.

Walnuts

- Walnuts are another great source of omega-3 fatty acids, as well as antioxidants and fiber. They can help lower inflammation and support heart health. Add walnuts to your diet by sprinkling them on salads, yogurt, or oatmeal, or by enjoying them as a snack.

Recipes Highlighting These Superfoods

Incorporating anti-inflammatory superfoods into your meals doesn't have to be complicated. Here are some simple and delicious recipes that highlight these powerful ingredients:

Turmeric Ginger Smoothie

- **Ingredients**: Fresh turmeric root, fresh ginger root, banana, mango, coconut milk, honey.
- **Preparation**: Blend all ingredients until smooth. Enjoy immediately for a refreshing and anti-inflammatory boost.

Blueberry Chia Pudding

- **Ingredients**: Chia seeds, almond milk, fresh blueberries, honey, vanilla extract.

- **Preparation**: Combine chia seeds, almond milk, honey, and vanilla extract in a bowl. Stir well and refrigerate overnight. In the morning, top with fresh blueberries and enjoy.

Baked Salmon with Lemon and Dill

- **Ingredients**: Salmon filets, olive oil, lemon slices, fresh dill, garlic, salt, and pepper.
- **Preparation**: Preheat oven to 375°F (190°C). Place salmon filets on a baking sheet lined with parchment paper. Drizzle with olive oil and season with salt and pepper. Top with lemon slices, fresh dill, and minced garlic. Bake for 20-25 minutes until salmon is cooked through.

Kale and Quinoa Salad

- **Ingredients**: Fresh kale, cooked quinoa, cherry tomatoes, cucumber, red onion, avocado, olive oil, lemon juice, salt, and pepper.
- **Preparation**: In a large bowl, massage kale with olive oil and lemon juice until softened. Add cooked quinoa, cherry tomatoes, cucumber, red

onion, and avocado. Toss to combine and season with salt and pepper.

Walnut and Berry Parfait

- **Ingredients**: Greek yogurt, fresh berries (blueberries, strawberries, raspberries), chopped walnuts, honey.
- **Preparation**: Layer Greek yogurt, fresh berries, and chopped walnuts in a glass. Drizzle with honey and enjoy it as a healthy breakfast or snack.

Balancing Macronutrients

Balancing macronutrients—proteins, fats, and carbohydrates—is essential for maintaining energy levels, supporting metabolic function, and reducing inflammation. Here's how to achieve a balanced intake of macronutrients with a focus on anti-inflammatory foods:

Proteins

- Choose lean protein sources such as chicken, turkey, fish, tofu, and legumes. Protein is crucial for building and repairing tissues, and it also plays a role in immune function. Aim to include a source of protein in every meal to keep you full and satisfied.

Fats

- Opt for healthy fats from sources like avocados, nuts, seeds, and olive oil. These fats help reduce inflammation and support brain and heart health. Avoid trans fats and limit saturated fats, which can increase inflammation.

Carbohydrates

- Focus on complex carbohydrates such as whole grains, fruits, and vegetables. These foods provide fiber, vitamins, and minerals that support overall health and help maintain stable blood sugar levels. Limit refined carbohydrates and sugars, which can cause spikes in blood sugar and contribute to inflammation.

Sample Balanced Meal:

Grilled Chicken with Quinoa and Roasted Vegetables

- **Ingredients**: Chicken breast, quinoa, mixed vegetables (such as bell peppers, zucchini, and carrots), olive oil, garlic, salt, and pepper.
- **Preparation**: Season chicken breast with olive oil, garlic, salt, and pepper. Grill until fully cooked. Cook quinoa according to package instructions. Roast mixed vegetables in the oven with olive oil, garlic, salt, and pepper until tender. Serve grilled chicken over a bed of quinoa with a side of roasted vegetables for a balanced and anti-inflammatory meal.

By incorporating these superfoods into your diet, following simple and nourishing recipes, and balancing your macronutrients, you can effectively build anti-inflammatory habits that support your health and well-being. These practices, established in Week 2, will create a solid foundation for continued success in managing inflammation and promoting overall health.

Mindful Eating Practices

Mindful eating practices play a crucial role in an anti-inflammatory diet, helping you develop a healthier relationship with food and promoting better digestion and overall well-being. By focusing on eating with intention, controlling portions, timing meals appropriately, and listening to your body's signals, you can enhance the benefits of your dietary choices and support your journey towards reduced inflammation and improved health.

Eating with Intention

Eating with intention means being fully present during your meals, paying attention to the flavors, textures, and aromas of your food. This practice encourages you to slow down and savor each bite, which can enhance your enjoyment of food and prevent overeating. When you eat with intention, you become more aware of what you are consuming, allowing you to make healthier choices and appreciate the nutritional value of your meals.

To eat with intention, start by eliminating distractions such as television, smartphones, or work-related activities during mealtime. Create a calm and pleasant eating environment, and focus solely on your food. Take small bites and chew thoroughly, allowing your taste buds to fully experience the flavors. This mindful approach to eating can improve digestion, as chewing thoroughly aids in breaking down food more effectively, making it easier for your body to absorb nutrients. Additionally, eating slowly gives your brain time to register feelings of fullness, helping you avoid overeating.

Portion Control and Meal Timing

Portion control and meal timing are essential aspects of mindful eating that can help regulate your body's inflammatory response and maintain stable energy levels throughout the day. Eating large portions can lead to overeating and weight gain, both of which are linked to increased inflammation. On the other hand, eating too little can leave you feeling unsatisfied and prone to unhealthy snacking. Finding the right balance is key to maintaining a healthy weight and reducing inflammation.

To practice portion control, start by using smaller plates and bowls, which can help you naturally eat smaller portions. Measure out serving sizes, especially for calorie-dense foods like nuts, seeds, and oils, to ensure you are not consuming too much. Listen to your body's hunger and fullness cues, and stop eating when you feel satisfied, not stuffed. Meal timing is also important for maintaining stable blood sugar levels and preventing inflammation. Aim to eat balanced meals and snacks at regular intervals throughout the day, ideally every 3-4 hours. This helps keep your energy levels steady and prevents overeating later in the day.

Listening to Your Body's Signals

Listening to your body's signals is a fundamental aspect of mindful eating that involves tuning into your hunger and fullness cues, as well as recognizing how different foods affect your body. By paying attention to these signals, you can better understand your body's needs and make dietary choices that support your health and well-being.

Hunger signals can vary from person to person, but common signs include a growling stomach, feeling lightheaded, or experiencing a dip in energy levels. Instead of eating out of habit or boredom, wait until you experience true hunger before starting a meal. Similarly, recognize when you are comfortably full and stop eating at that point. Eating beyond fullness can lead to discomfort and digestive issues, which can contribute to inflammation.

In addition to hunger and fullness cues, pay attention to how different foods make you feel. Some foods may leave you feeling energized and satisfied, while others might cause bloating, fatigue, or other digestive issues. Keeping a food diary can help you track these reactions and identify any patterns or sensitivities. By listening to your body's signals, you can make informed decisions about what foods work best for you and adjust your diet accordingly.

Mindful eating practices such as eating with intention, practicing portion control and proper meal timing, and listening to your body's signals are essential for maintaining a healthy anti-inflammatory diet. These practices not only enhance your enjoyment of food but also support better digestion, stable energy levels, and overall well-being. By incorporating mindful eating into your daily routine, you can foster a healthier relationship with food and promote long-term health and vitality.

Chapter 6: Week 3 – Enhancing Gut Health

Gut health is a fundamental aspect of overall well-being and plays a crucial role in managing inflammation. A balanced gut microbiome supports digestion, nutrient absorption, and immune function, all of which are essential for maintaining a healthy body. During Week 3, the focus shifts to enhancing gut health by incorporating probiotics and prebiotics into your diet. These beneficial compounds help cultivate a diverse and thriving gut microbiome, which can significantly reduce inflammation and improve overall health. This chapter explores foods that support a healthy gut, the benefits of fermented foods, and provides recipe ideas to help you integrate these foods into your daily meals.

Probiotics and Prebiotics

Probiotics and prebiotics are key players in maintaining a healthy gut microbiome. Probiotics are live beneficial bacteria that help populate the gut with healthy microbes, while prebiotics are non-digestible fibers that serve as food for these beneficial bacteria. Together, they create a balanced environment that supports optimal gut function and reduces inflammation.

Foods That Support a Healthy Gut Microbiome

Several foods are rich in probiotics and prebiotics, and incorporating them into your diet can help enhance gut health. Probiotic-rich foods include:

- **Yogurt**: Look for plain, unsweetened yogurt with live and active cultures.
- **Kefir**: A fermented milk drink that contains a variety of beneficial bacteria and yeasts.
- **Sauerkraut**: Fermented cabbage that is rich in probiotics and enzymes.
- **Kimchi**: A spicy Korean side dish made from fermented vegetables.
- **Miso**: A fermented soybean paste used in Japanese cuisine.
- **Tempeh**: A fermented soybean product that is a good source of protein and probiotics.

Prebiotic-rich foods include:

- **Garlic**: Contains inulin, a type of prebiotic fiber.
- **Onions**: Also rich in inulin and other prebiotic fibers.
- **Asparagus**: A good source of inulin and other prebiotics.
- **Bananas**: Contain resistant starch and other prebiotic fibers.
- **Leeks**: High in prebiotic fibers like inulin.
- **Chicory root:** Often used as a coffee substitute, rich in inulin.

Fermented Foods and Their Benefits

Fermented foods are particularly beneficial for gut health because they contain live cultures that can help replenish and diversify the gut microbiome. Fermentation not only enhances the nutritional value of foods but also makes them easier to digest. The beneficial bacteria produced during fermentation can help improve gut health, boost the immune system, and reduce inflammation.

For example, yogurt and kefir are rich in probiotics that can help balance the gut microbiome and improve digestion. Sauerkraut and kimchi are excellent sources of lactic acid bacteria, which can enhance gut health and support immune function. Miso and tempeh provide both probiotics and valuable nutrients like vitamins and minerals, making them versatile additions to a healthy diet.

Recipe Ideas to Incorporate These Foods

Incorporating probiotic and prebiotic foods into your diet can be both delicious and straightforward. Here are some recipe ideas to help you get started:

Probiotic-Rich Recipes

1. Yogurt Parfait with Fresh Berries and Nuts

- **Ingredients**: Plain yogurt, fresh berries (such as blueberries, strawberries, or raspberries), chopped nuts (such as almonds or walnuts), honey (optional).

- **Preparation**: Layer plain yogurt with fresh berries and chopped nuts in a glass or bowl. Drizzle with honey if desired.

2. Kefir Smoothie

- **Ingredients**: Plain kefir, frozen berries, banana, spinach, chia seeds.
- **Preparation**: Blend all ingredients until smooth. Serve immediately.

3. Kimchi Fried Rice

- **Ingredients**: Cooked brown rice, kimchi, diced vegetables (such as carrots, bell peppers, and peas), sesame oil, soy sauce or tamari, green onions, sesame seeds.
- **Preparation**: Heat sesame oil in a pan and sauté diced vegetables until tender. Add cooked brown rice and kimchi, stirring to combine. Season with soy sauce or tamari. Garnish with green onions and sesame seeds before serving.

Prebiotic-Rich Recipes

1. Garlic and Asparagus Stir-Fry

- **Ingredients**: Fresh asparagus, minced garlic, olive oil, salt, and pepper.
- **Preparation**: Heat olive oil in a pan and sauté minced garlic until fragrant. Add asparagus and cook until tender. Season with salt and pepper.

2. Banana and Oat Breakfast Muffins

- **Ingredients**: Ripe bananas, rolled oats, almond flour, baking powder, eggs, honey, vanilla extract, chopped walnuts.
- **Preparation**: Preheat oven to 350°F (175°C). Mash bananas in a bowl and mix with rolled oats, almond flour, baking powder, eggs, honey, and vanilla extract. Fold in chopped walnuts. Divide batter into muffin tins and bake for 20-25 minutes.

3. Leek and Potato Soup

- **Ingredients**: Leeks, potatoes, vegetable broth, olive oil, garlic, salt, and pepper.
- **Preparation**: Sauté sliced leeks and minced garlic in olive oil until softened. Add diced potatoes and vegetable broth. Bring to a boil, then simmer until potatoes are tender. Blend until smooth and season with salt and pepper.

By incorporating these probiotic and prebiotic-rich foods into your diet, you can enhance your gut health and reduce inflammation. The recipes provided are simple, nutritious, and delicious, making it easy to enjoy the benefits of a healthy gut microbiome. As you continue your anti-inflammatory journey, maintaining a focus on gut health will support your overall well-being and help you achieve lasting results.

Reducing Inflammatory Triggers

Identifying and eliminating inflammatory triggers is a crucial step in managing chronic inflammation and enhancing overall health. Certain foods and substances can exacerbate inflammation in the body, leading to various health issues and discomfort. By pinpointing and removing these triggers, you can significantly reduce inflammation and improve your well-being. This section will guide you through the process of identifying potential food sensitivities, keeping a detailed food diary, and adjusting your diet based on your observations.

Identifying and Eliminating Potential Food Sensitivities

Food sensitivities and intolerances can cause chronic inflammation and a range of symptoms, from digestive issues and skin problems to headaches and joint pain. Unlike food allergies, which trigger an immediate immune response, food sensitivities can cause delayed reactions, making them harder to identify. Common culprits include gluten, dairy, soy, corn, eggs, and certain food additives.

To identify potential food sensitivities, start by eliminating the most common inflammatory foods from your diet for a period of two to four weeks. This elimination phase allows your body to reset and can help alleviate symptoms caused by these foods. During this time, focus on eating a variety of whole, unprocessed foods such as fruits, vegetables, lean proteins, and healthy fats. After the elimination period, gradually reintroduce the eliminated foods one at a time, allowing several days between each reintroduction to monitor for any adverse reactions. Pay attention to symptoms such as bloating, gas, skin rashes, headaches, and fatigue, which may indicate a sensitivity.

Keeping a Food Diary

Keeping a detailed food diary is an invaluable tool in identifying food sensitivities and understanding how different foods affect your body. By recording everything you eat and drink, along with any symptoms you experience, you can spot patterns and make connections between your diet and your health.

In your food diary, include the following information:

- **Foods and Beverages Consumed:** List all meals, snacks, and drinks, including portion sizes and ingredients.

- **Time of Consumption:** Note the time you ate or drank each item.

- **Symptoms**: Record any symptoms you experience, including their severity and timing relative to food consumption.

- **Other Factors**: Include other factors that might affect your health, such as stress levels, physical activity, sleep quality, and environmental exposures.

Review your food diary regularly to identify trends and correlations. For example, if you notice that you frequently experience digestive discomfort after consuming dairy products, this could indicate a sensitivity to lactose or casein. By systematically recording and analyzing your food intake and symptoms, you can gain insights into which foods might be contributing to inflammation and other health issues.

Adjusting Your Diet Based on Observations

Once you have identified potential food sensitivities through the elimination diet and food diary, the next step is to adjust your diet accordingly. Eliminating or reducing the consumption of problematic foods can significantly reduce inflammation and improve your overall health.

To adjust your diet:

- **Permanently Remove Identified Triggers:** If certain foods consistently cause adverse reactions, consider eliminating them from your diet permanently or significantly reducing your intake. For example, if gluten triggers symptoms, opt for gluten-free grains like quinoa, rice, and buckwheat.

- **Seek Alternatives:** Replace inflammatory foods with healthier alternatives. For instance, use almond milk or coconut milk instead of dairy milk, and choose olive oil or avocado oil instead of processed vegetable oils.

- **Balance Your Diet:** Ensure your diet remains balanced and nutrient-dense despite the elimination of certain foods. Include a variety of fruits, vegetables, lean proteins, healthy fats, and whole grains to meet your nutritional needs.

- **Monitor and Adjust:** Continue to monitor your symptoms and dietary intake, making further adjustments as needed. Your body's response to foods can change over time, so remain attentive and adaptable.

Additionally, consider seeking guidance from a healthcare professional or a registered dietitian, especially if you have multiple food sensitivities or complex dietary needs. They can help you create a tailored eating plan that supports your health while avoiding inflammatory triggers.

Reducing inflammatory triggers involves identifying and eliminating potential food sensitivities, keeping a detailed food diary, and adjusting your diet based on your observations. By taking these steps, you can significantly reduce inflammation, alleviate symptoms, and enhance your overall health and well-being.

Chapter 7: Week 4 – Long-Term Sustainability

As you approach the end of your 30-day anti-inflammatory diet journey, the focus shifts to maintaining these healthy habits for the long term. Achieving long-term sustainability involves transitioning from a strict dietary plan to a flexible lifestyle that incorporates anti-inflammatory principles. This chapter will guide you through this transition, offering strategies for dining out and handling special occasions, and emphasizing the importance of continuing education and staying motivated. By embedding these practices into your daily life, you can ensure lasting benefits and a healthier, inflammation-free future.

Maintaining Anti-Inflammatory Habits

Transitioning from a strict plan to a flexible lifestyle is crucial for sustaining the progress you have made. During the initial phase, you likely followed a structured diet with specific guidelines and meal plans. As you move forward, the goal is to integrate these habits into a more adaptable approach that fits your lifestyle while still prioritizing anti-inflammatory foods and practices.

Transitioning from a Strict Plan to a Flexible Lifestyle

The key to a successful transition is to retain the core principles of your anti-inflammatory diet while allowing for greater flexibility. This means continuing to prioritize whole, nutrient-dense foods, but also giving yourself permission to enjoy occasional treats and indulgences in moderation. Here are some tips for making this transition smoothly:

1. **Gradual Integration:** Slowly reintroduce foods you may have restricted during the initial phase, paying attention to how they affect your body. This helps you understand your tolerance levels and make informed choices.

2. **Flexible Meal Planning:** Instead of following a rigid meal plan, create a weekly framework that allows for variety and spontaneity. Focus on

balancing macronutrients and including a variety of anti-inflammatory foods in each meal.

3. **Mindful Eating:** Continue practicing mindful eating to maintain a healthy relationship with food. Pay attention to your hunger and fullness cues, and enjoy your meals without distraction.

4. **Routine Adjustments:** Adapt your eating habits to fit your lifestyle. If you have a busy schedule, prepare meals and snacks in advance to ensure you always have healthy options available.

Strategies for Dining Out and Special Occasions

Dining out and special occasions can be challenging when trying to maintain an anti-inflammatory diet, but with some strategies in place, you can enjoy these experiences without compromising your health goals.

1. **Plan Ahead:** Before dining out, check the restaurant's menu online to identify healthy, anti-inflammatory options. Look for dishes that include plenty of vegetables, lean proteins, and healthy fats.

2. **Ask Questions:** Don't hesitate to ask the waiter about how dishes are prepared and request modifications to make them healthier. For example, ask for grilled instead of fried, or for dressing on the side.

3. **Portion Control**: Restaurant portions are often larger than necessary. Consider sharing a meal or taking half of it home to avoid overeating.

4. **Focus on Enjoyment:** Remember that social occasions are about more than just food. Focus on enjoying the company and the experience, and allow yourself to indulge moderately without guilt.

5. **Bring a Dish:** If you're attending a potluck or party, consider bringing a healthy, anti-inflammatory dish that you enjoy. This ensures there's at least one option that fits your dietary needs.

Continuing Education and Staying Motivated

Continuing education and staying motivated are essential for maintaining long-term dietary habits. As new research emerges and your body's needs change, keeping yourself informed and inspired can help you stay on track.

1. **Stay Informed:** Keep up-to-date with the latest research on nutrition and inflammation. Subscribe to reputable health newsletters, read books, and follow experts in the field. This ongoing education helps you make informed decisions and adapt your diet as needed.

2. **Set New Goals:** Regularly set new health goals to keep yourself motivated. These goals can be related to fitness, weight management, or even learning new healthy recipes. Having something to work towards can keep you engaged and focused.

3. **Build a Support Network:** Surround yourself with supportive friends and family who understand and respect your health goals. Joining

a community, either online or in person, can provide additional motivation and accountability.

4. **Celebrate Progress:** Acknowledge and celebrate your achievements, no matter how small. Reflect on how far you've come since starting your anti-inflammatory journey and use that progress as motivation to continue.

5. **Listen to Your Body:** Pay attention to how your body responds to different foods and activities. Adjust your diet and lifestyle based on what makes you feel your best, and be flexible in your approach.

Maintaining anti-inflammatory habits involves transitioning from a strict plan to a flexible lifestyle, implementing strategies for dining out and special occasions, and continuing education and motivation. By embedding these practices into your daily routine, you can enjoy a balanced, sustainable approach to eating that supports long-term health and reduces inflammation. The final sections of this book will offer additional resources, tips, and recipes to help you continue your journey towards a healthier, more vibrant life.

Balancing Nutrition with Lifestyle Choices

Balancing nutrition with lifestyle choices is essential for optimizing your health and managing chronic inflammation. While diet plays a crucial role in reducing inflammation, other factors such as physical activity, stress management, and sleep are equally important. A holistic approach that integrates these elements can help you achieve and maintain long-term health and well-being. This section explores the importance of incorporating physical activity, effective stress management techniques, and prioritizing sleep and recovery.

Incorporating Physical Activity

Regular physical activity is a cornerstone of a healthy lifestyle and has significant anti-inflammatory benefits. Exercise helps regulate the body's inflammatory response, reduces the risk of chronic diseases, and improves overall physical and mental health. Here's how to incorporate physical activity into your routine:

1. **Find Activities You Enjoy:** Choose exercises that you find enjoyable and sustainable, whether it's walking, cycling, swimming, yoga, or dancing. Enjoyable activities are more likely to become long-term habits.

2. **Aim for Consistency:** Aim to engage in moderate-intensity physical activity for at least 150 minutes per week, as recommended by health guidelines. This can be broken down into 30 minutes a day, five days a week.

3. **Incorporate Variety:** Include a mix of cardiovascular exercises, strength training, and flexibility exercises to promote overall fitness. This variety helps prevent boredom and works different muscle groups.

4. **Listen to Your Body:** Pay attention to how your body responds to exercise. Start slowly and gradually increase the intensity and duration of

your workouts. Rest and recover when needed to prevent injury and overtraining.

Regular physical activity not only helps reduce inflammation but also boosts mood, enhances energy levels, and supports weight management. It is a vital component of a holistic approach to health.

Stress Management Techniques

Chronic stress is a major contributor to inflammation and can negatively impact your health in numerous ways. Effective stress management techniques can help you maintain a balanced inflammatory response and improve overall well-being. Here are some strategies to manage stress:

1. **Mindfulness and Meditation:** Practicing mindfulness and meditation can help reduce stress and promote relaxation. Techniques such as deep breathing, guided imagery, and progressive muscle relaxation can calm the mind and body.

2. **Physical Activity:** Exercise is a natural stress reliever that releases endorphins, the body's feel-good hormones. Activities like yoga and tai chi combine physical movement with mindfulness, providing dual benefits.

3. **Healthy Social Connections:** Maintaining strong social connections with family and friends provides emotional support and can reduce stress. Make time for meaningful interactions and activities you enjoy with loved ones.

4. **Time Management:** Effective time management can help reduce stress by allowing you to prioritize tasks and manage your workload more efficiently. Break tasks into manageable steps, set realistic goals, and take regular breaks.

5. **Hobbies and Leisure Activities:** Engaging in hobbies and leisure activities that you enjoy can provide a mental break from daily stressors. Whether it's reading, gardening, painting, or playing an instrument, find activities that bring you joy.

Incorporating these stress management techniques into your daily routine can help you maintain a calm and balanced state, reducing the impact of stress on your health.

The Importance of Sleep and Recovery

Sleep and recovery are critical for maintaining a healthy immune system and reducing inflammation. Quality sleep allows the body to repair and regenerate, supporting overall health and well-being. Here's why sleep and recovery are important and how to prioritize them:

1. **Restorative Sleep:** Aim for 7-9 hours of quality sleep per night. Sleep is essential for cellular repair, immune function, and hormonal balance. Chronic sleep deprivation can lead to increased inflammation and a higher risk of chronic diseases.

2. **Establish a Sleep Routine:** Create a consistent sleep schedule by going to bed and waking up at the same time every day, even on weekends. This

helps regulate your body's internal clock and improves sleep quality.

3. **Create a Sleep-Friendly Environment:** Ensure your bedroom is conducive to sleep. Keep the room cool, dark, and quiet, and invest in a comfortable mattress and pillows. Avoid screens and electronic devices at least an hour before bedtime, as the blue light can interfere with sleep.

4. **Relaxation Techniques:** Practice relaxation techniques before bed to promote restful sleep. This could include reading, taking a warm bath, or listening to calming music. Avoid caffeine and heavy meals close to bedtime.

5. **Prioritize Recovery:** In addition to sleep, incorporate rest and recovery into your physical activity routine. Allow time for your muscles to recover between workouts, and include rest days to prevent overtraining and injury.

By prioritizing sleep and recovery, you can support your body's natural healing processes and maintain a healthy inflammatory response. Quality sleep and adequate rest are essential for sustaining energy levels, cognitive function, and overall health.

Balancing nutrition with lifestyle choices involves incorporating regular physical activity, implementing effective stress management techniques, and prioritizing sleep and recovery. By adopting a holistic approach that integrates these elements, you can enhance your overall well-being, reduce inflammation, and achieve long-term health and vitality. This comprehensive strategy supports not only your physical health but also your mental and emotional well-being, contributing to a balanced and fulfilling life.

Chapter 8: Recipes for a Lifetime

In this chapter, we provide a collection of recipes designed to become staples in your diet, supporting your anti-inflammatory journey for years to come. These recipes are not only delicious but also packed with nutrients that help reduce inflammation and promote overall health. This section focuses on breakfasts, with a particular emphasis on anti-inflammatory smoothie bowls and other nutritious, filling options that will start your day on the right note.

Breakfasts

Breakfast is a crucial meal that sets the tone for your day. Eating a nutrient-dense, anti-inflammatory breakfast can help stabilize your blood sugar levels, provide sustained energy, and support overall health. Here are some delicious and healthy breakfast ideas to incorporate into your daily routine.

Anti-Inflammatory Smoothie Bowls

Smoothie bowls are a fantastic way to pack a variety of anti-inflammatory ingredients into one meal. They are versatile, easy to make, and can be customized to suit your taste preferences and nutritional needs. Here are a few recipes to get you started:

1. Berry Bliss Smoothie Bowl

Ingredients:

- 1 cup frozen mixed berries (blueberries, strawberries, raspberries)
- 1 banana
- 1/2 cup unsweetened almond milk
- 1 tablespoon chia seeds
- 1 tablespoon almond butter
- Toppings: fresh berries, sliced banana, granola, and a drizzle of honey

Preparation:

- Blend the frozen berries, banana, almond milk, chia seeds, and almond butter until smooth.

- Pour into a bowl and add your favorite toppings.

2. Tropical Turmeric Smoothie Bowl

Ingredients:

- 1 cup frozen mango chunks
- 1/2 cup frozen pineapple chunks
- 1 banana
- 1/2 cup coconut water
- 1 teaspoon turmeric powder
- 1/2 teaspoon fresh ginger, grated
- Toppings: shredded coconut, sliced kiwi, chia seeds, and goji berries
- Preparation:
- Blend the mango, pineapple, banana, coconut water, turmeric, and ginger until smooth.
- Pour into a bowl and add your favorite toppings.

3. Green Detox Smoothie Bowl

Ingredients:

- 1 cup spinach
- 1/2 avocado

- 1 banana

- 1/2 cup unsweetened almond milk

- 1 tablespoon flaxseeds

- 1 tablespoon protein powder (optional)

- Toppings: sliced almonds, fresh berries, and a sprinkle of hemp seeds

Preparation:

- Blend the spinach, avocado, banana, almond milk, flaxseeds, and protein powder until smooth.

- Pour into a bowl and add your favorite toppings.

Nutritious and Filling Options

For those who prefer a heartier breakfast, here are some nutritious and filling options that are easy to prepare and rich in anti-inflammatory ingredients:

1. Overnight Oats with Berries and Nuts

Ingredients:

- 1/2 cup rolled oats

- 1/2 cup unsweetened almond milk

- 1 tablespoon chia seeds
- 1/2 teaspoon cinnamon
- 1/2 cup fresh or frozen berries
- 1 tablespoon chopped nuts (such as almonds or walnuts)
- Drizzle of honey (optional)

Preparation:

- Combine the oats, almond milk, chia seeds, and cinnamon in a jar or bowl.
- Stir well and refrigerate overnight.
- In the morning, top with berries, nuts, and a drizzle of honey.

2. Quinoa Breakfast Bowl

Ingredients:

- 1/2 cup cooked quinoa
- 1/4 cup unsweetened almond milk
- 1/2 banana, sliced
- 1 tablespoon almond butter
- 1 tablespoon hemp seeds

- 1/2 teaspoon cinnamon

- Fresh berries for topping

Preparation:

- In a bowl, combine cooked quinoa and almond milk.

- Top with banana slices, almond butter, hemp seeds, and cinnamon.

- Add fresh berries on top and enjoy.

3. Avocado Toast with Turmeric and Poached Egg

Ingredients:

- 1 slice whole-grain bread, toasted

- 1/2 ripe avocado

- 1 poached egg

- 1/4 teaspoon turmeric powder

- Salt and pepper to taste

- Red pepper flakes (optional)

Preparation:

- Mash the avocado and spread it on the toasted bread.
- Sprinkle with turmeric powder, salt, and pepper.
- Top with a poached egg and a sprinkle of red pepper flakes for an extra kick.

4. Chia Pudding with Fresh Fruit

Ingredients:

- 1/4 cup chia seeds
- 1 cup unsweetened almond milk
- 1 teaspoon vanilla extract
- Fresh fruit for topping (such as berries, mango, or kiwi)

Preparation:

- In a jar or bowl, combine chia seeds, almond milk, and vanilla extract.
- Stir well and refrigerate for at least 4 hours or overnight.
- In the morning, top with fresh fruit and enjoy.

By incorporating these anti-inflammatory breakfast recipes into your daily routine, you can start each day with a nutritious, satisfying meal that supports your health and well-being. These recipes are easy to prepare, delicious, and packed with ingredients that help reduce inflammation and provide sustained energy throughout the day.

Lunches and Dinners

Balanced meals rich in anti-inflammatory ingredients are essential for sustaining energy, supporting overall health, and reducing inflammation throughout the day. Lunch and dinner provide opportunities to incorporate a variety of nutrient-dense foods that can help maintain a balanced diet. This section offers easy-to-follow recipes that are both delicious and beneficial for your health.

Balanced Meals Rich in Anti-Inflammatory Ingredients

Creating balanced meals involves combining lean proteins, healthy fats, and plenty of fruits and vegetables.

These components provide the necessary nutrients to fight inflammation and support overall wellness.

Grilled Chicken and Vegetable Quinoa Bowl

Ingredients:

- 1 cup cooked quinoa
- 1 grilled chicken breast, sliced
- 1 cup mixed vegetables (such as bell peppers, zucchini, and cherry tomatoes)
- 1/4 cup hummus
- 1 tablespoon olive oil
- Juice of 1 lemon
- Salt and pepper to taste

Preparation:

- Toss the mixed vegetables in olive oil, salt, and pepper, then grill or roast them until tender.
- Combine the cooked quinoa, grilled chicken, and vegetables in a bowl.
- Drizzle with lemon juice and add a dollop of hummus on top.

Turmeric and Ginger Salmon with Steamed Broccoli

Ingredients:

- 2 salmon filets
- 1 teaspoon turmeric powder
- 1 teaspoon grated fresh ginger
- 2 tablespoons olive oil
- 1 lemon, sliced
- 2 cups broccoli florets
- Salt and pepper to taste

Preparation:

- Preheat the oven to 375°F (190°C).
- Mix turmeric, ginger, olive oil, salt, and pepper in a small bowl.
- Rub the mixture over the salmon filets and place them on a baking sheet.
- Top with lemon slices and bake for 20-25 minutes, or until the salmon is cooked through.
- Steam the broccoli until tender and serve alongside the salmon.

Chickpea and Spinach Curry

Ingredients:

- 1 can chickpeas, drained and rinsed
- 2 cups fresh spinach
- 1 onion, chopped
- 2 garlic cloves, minced
- 1 tablespoon grated ginger
- 1 can coconut milk
- 2 tablespoons curry powder
- 1 tablespoon olive oil
- Salt and pepper to taste

Preparation:

- Heat olive oil in a large pan over medium heat. Add the onion, garlic, and ginger, and sauté until fragrant.
- Stir in the curry powder and cook for another minute.
- Add the chickpeas and coconut milk, bringing the mixture to a simmer.

- Stir in the spinach and cook until wilted. Season with salt and pepper to taste.
- Serve over brown rice or quinoa.

Easy-to-Follow Recipes

Here are a few more easy-to-follow recipes that are rich in anti-inflammatory ingredients and perfect for lunch or dinner:

Quinoa and Black Bean Stuffed Peppers

Ingredients:

- 4 large bell peppers, halved and seeds removed
- 1 cup cooked quinoa
- 1 can black beans, drained and rinsed
- 1 cup corn kernels
- 1 can diced tomatoes
- 1 teaspoon cumin
- 1 teaspoon chili powder
- 1/2 cup shredded cheese (optional)
- Salt and pepper to taste

Preparation:

- Preheat the oven to 375°F (190°C).
- Mix quinoa, black beans, corn, diced tomatoes, cumin, chili powder, salt, and pepper in a large bowl.
- Stuff the bell pepper halves with the quinoa mixture and place them in a baking dish.
- Top with shredded cheese if desired.
- Bake for 25-30 minutes, or until the peppers are tender.

Lentil and Vegetable Stir-Fry

Ingredients:

- 1 cup cooked lentils
- 1 cup mixed vegetables (such as bell peppers, carrots, and snap peas)
- 2 tablespoons soy sauce or tamari
- 1 tablespoon sesame oil
- 2 garlic cloves, minced
- 1 teaspoon grated fresh ginger
- 1 tablespoon sesame seeds

- 2 green onions, chopped

Preparation:

- Heat sesame oil in a large pan over medium-high heat.
- Add the garlic and ginger, sautéing until fragrant.
- Add the mixed vegetables and stir-fry until tender-crisp.
- Stir in the cooked lentils and soy sauce, cooking until heated through.
- Sprinkle it with sesame seeds and green onions before serving.

Snacks and Desserts

Healthy snacks and guilt-free desserts are important for maintaining energy levels between meals and satisfying your sweet tooth without compromising your anti-inflammatory goals. This section provides a variety of options that are both nutritious and delicious.

Healthy Snacks to Keep Inflammation at Bay

Apple Slices with Almond Butter

Ingredients:

- 1 apple, sliced
- 2 tablespoons almond butter
- Preparation:
- Spread almond butter on apple slices for a simple and nutritious snack.

Greek Yogurt with Berries and Honey

Ingredients:

- 1 cup plain Greek yogurt
- 1/2 cup fresh berries (such as blueberries, raspberries, or strawberries)
- 1 tablespoon honey

Preparation:

- Top Greek yogurt with fresh berries and a drizzle of honey.

Vegetable Crudités with Hummus

Ingredients:

- Assorted fresh vegetables (such as carrots, cucumber, bell peppers, and celery), sliced
- 1/2 cup hummus

Preparation:

- Arrange vegetable slices on a plate and serve with hummus for dipping.

Guilt-Free Desserts

Chia Seed Pudding

Ingredients:

- 1/4 cup chia seeds
- 1 cup unsweetened almond milk
- 1 teaspoon vanilla extract
- 1 tablespoon honey or maple syrup
- Fresh fruit for topping

Preparation:

- In a bowl, combine chia seeds, almond milk, vanilla extract, and honey.
- Stir well and refrigerate for at least 4 hours or overnight.
- Top with fresh fruit before serving.

Dark Chocolate Avocado Mousse

Ingredients:

- 2 ripe avocados
- 1/4 cup unsweetened cocoa powder
- 1/4 cup maple syrup
- 1 teaspoon vanilla extract
- Pinch of sea salt

Preparation:

- Blend all ingredients until smooth and creamy.
- Chill in the refrigerator for at least 30 minutes before serving.

Baked Apples with Cinnamon and Walnuts

Ingredients:

- 4 apples, cored
- 1/4 cup chopped walnuts
- 2 tablespoons honey
- 1 teaspoon cinnamon
- 1/4 teaspoon nutmeg

Preparation:

- Preheat the oven to 350°F (175°C).
- Place the cored apples in a baking dish.
- In a small bowl, mix chopped walnuts, honey, cinnamon, and nutmeg.
- Stuff the mixture into the center of each apple.
- Bake for 20-25 minutes, or until the apples are tender.

By incorporating these lunches, dinners, snacks, and desserts into your diet, you can enjoy a wide variety of delicious and nutritious meals that help keep inflammation at bay. These recipes are easy to prepare and full of anti-inflammatory ingredients, making them perfect for supporting your long-term health goals.

Chapter 9: Success Stories and Testimonials

One of the most inspiring aspects of embarking on an anti-inflammatory diet journey is hearing about the real-life transformations of others who have successfully adopted these principles. Success stories and testimonials provide motivation, encouragement, and practical insights for anyone looking to make similar changes. This chapter shares the experiences of individuals who followed the anti-inflammatory diet plan, highlighting their before and after experiences, and offering tips and advice for achieving lasting success.

Real-Life Transformations

The transformative power of an anti-inflammatory diet can be seen in the diverse stories of individuals who have experienced significant improvements in their health and quality of life. These real-life transformations illustrate the profound impact that dietary changes can have on managing chronic inflammation and promoting overall well-being.

John's Journey to Pain-Free Living

John, a 52-year-old engineer, struggled with chronic joint pain and stiffness due to arthritis. Despite trying various medications and treatments, his symptoms persisted, affecting his ability to work and enjoy recreational activities. After learning about the anti-inflammatory diet, John decided to give it a try. Within a few weeks, he noticed a reduction in pain and inflammation. Over the next few months, his mobility improved, and he was able to resume activities like hiking and playing tennis. John's transformation underscores the importance of dietary choices in managing chronic conditions and improving quality of life.

Sarah's Success in Managing Autoimmune Symptoms

Sarah, a 34-year-old teacher, was diagnosed with an autoimmune disorder that caused fatigue, digestive issues, and skin rashes. Frustrated with the lack of progress using conventional treatments, Sarah turned to the anti-inflammatory diet. By eliminating trigger foods and incorporating nutrient-dense, anti-inflammatory ingredients, she experienced a significant reduction in her symptoms. Her energy levels increased, her digestive issues resolved, and her skin cleared up. Sarah's story highlights the potential of dietary interventions to complement medical treatments and achieve better health outcomes.

Stories from Individuals Who Followed the Plan

Hearing from individuals who have followed the anti-inflammatory diet plan can provide valuable insights and inspiration. These stories demonstrate the practical application of the diet and the diverse benefits it can offer.

Mike's Weight Loss and Improved Health Markers

Mike, a 45-year-old accountant, struggled with obesity and related health issues, including high blood pressure and elevated cholesterol levels. Motivated to improve his health, Mike adopted the anti-inflammatory diet. Over the course of a year, he lost 50 pounds and saw significant improvements in his health markers. His blood pressure normalized, his cholesterol levels dropped, and he felt more energetic and focused. Mike's story illustrates how the anti-inflammatory diet can support weight loss and improve overall health.

Laura's Enhanced Mental Clarity and Mood

Laura, a 29-year-old marketing professional, experienced frequent mood swings, brain fog, and anxiety. After learning about the link between diet and mental health, she decided to try the anti-inflammatory diet. Within a few weeks, Laura noticed enhanced mental clarity, improved mood stability, and reduced anxiety. Her productivity at work increased, and she felt more balanced and positive in her daily life. Laura's experience shows the connection between diet and mental well-being and how dietary changes can enhance cognitive and emotional health.

Before and After Experiences

The before and after experiences of individuals who have adopted the anti-inflammatory diet provide compelling evidence of its effectiveness. These transformations often involve significant improvements in physical, mental, and emotional health.

David's Cardiovascular Health Improvement

Before adopting the anti-inflammatory diet, David, a 60-year-old retired firefighter, faced multiple cardiovascular issues, including hypertension and high triglycerides. His doctor recommended dietary changes as part of his treatment plan. After six months on the anti-inflammatory diet, David's blood pressure stabilized, and his triglyceride levels dropped significantly. He also experienced increased energy levels and better overall health. David's before and after experience emphasizes the diet's potential to improve heart health and prevent cardiovascular diseases.

Emma's Skin Transformation

Emma, a 25-year-old graphic designer, dealt with chronic acne and eczema that affected her confidence and social interactions. She decided to try the anti-inflammatory diet to address these skin issues from the inside out. After three months, Emma saw a remarkable improvement in her skin. Her acne cleared up, and her eczema flare-ups became less frequent and severe. Emma's transformation highlights the impact of diet on skin health and the importance of internal factors in achieving clear, healthy skin.

Tips and Advice from Those Who Succeeded

Individuals who have successfully followed the anti-inflammatory diet often have valuable tips and advice to share. Their insights can help others navigate the journey more effectively and achieve lasting results.

Consistency is Key

Many individuals emphasize the importance of consistency in following the anti-inflammatory diet.

Making gradual, sustainable changes and sticking to the plan, even when it's challenging, is crucial for long-term success. Consistency helps build healthy habits and allows the body to adjust and respond positively to the dietary changes.

Listen to Your Body

Listening to your body and paying attention to how different foods affect you is another common piece of advice. Keeping a food diary and tracking symptoms can help identify trigger foods and better understand your body's unique responses. Adjusting the diet based on personal experiences and needs ensures it remains effective and tailored to individual health goals.

Stay Educated and Informed

Continuing to educate yourself about nutrition and staying informed about the latest research can help maintain motivation and make informed choices. Reading books, following reputable health websites, and seeking guidance from healthcare professionals can provide valuable insights and keep you engaged in your health journey.

Seek Support

Having a support system can make a significant difference in staying committed to the diet. Sharing your goals with friends and family, joining support groups, or finding an accountability partner can provide encouragement, motivation, and a sense of community. Support from others who understand your journey can help you stay on track and overcome challenges.

Celebrate Progress

Celebrating progress, no matter how small, is essential for maintaining motivation. Recognize and reward yourself for the positive changes and improvements you experience. Celebrating milestones can boost confidence and reinforce the benefits of the anti-inflammatory diet, encouraging continued adherence and success.

The success stories and testimonials of individuals who have followed the anti-inflammatory diet provide powerful motivation and practical insights. Their real-life transformations, before and after experiences, and valuable tips and advice can inspire and guide you on your own journey towards better health and reduced inflammation. By learning from their experiences, you can achieve lasting success and enjoy the many benefits of a healthier, more balanced lifestyle.

Conclusion

As you reach the conclusion of this book, it is important to reflect on the journey you have undertaken and the progress you have made. Adopting an anti-inflammatory diet and lifestyle is a transformative process that involves not just changes in eating habits but also shifts in mindset and overall wellness practices. The journey ahead is about maintaining these positive changes, continuing to learn and grow, and sharing your experiences to inspire others.

The Journey Ahead

The journey ahead involves integrating the knowledge and practices you have gained into your daily life. This is not just a 30-day plan but a lifelong commitment to health and well-being. The benefits you have experienced so far—from reduced inflammation and improved energy levels to better mental clarity and overall health—are just the beginning. As you move forward, it is essential to maintain these habits and remain proactive in your health journey.

Reflecting on Your Progress

Take a moment to reflect on your progress. Consider the changes you have made and the improvements you have noticed in your health and well-being. Reflecting on your journey can help you appreciate how far you have come and reinforce the positive impact of your efforts.

- **Physical Changes:** Notice any physical changes such as weight loss, reduced joint pain, improved skin condition, and increased energy levels. These tangible benefits are a testament to the effectiveness of the anti-inflammatory diet.

- **Mental and Emotional Well-being:** Reflect on improvements in mental clarity, mood stability, and overall emotional well-being. These aspects are equally important as physical health and contribute to a holistic sense of wellness.

- **Habits and Mindset:** Acknowledge the new habits you have formed and the mindset shifts you have experienced. These changes are foundational for sustaining a healthy lifestyle.

By recognizing and celebrating your progress, you can stay motivated and committed to your health goals.

Continuing Your Health Journey

Continuing your health journey involves staying informed, adapting to new challenges, and remaining flexible in your approach. Here are some strategies to help you stay on track:

- **Ongoing Education:** Keep learning about nutrition, wellness, and the latest research on inflammation and health. Stay curious and open-minded, and seek out reliable sources of information to deepen your understanding.
- **Adapting to Changes:** Life is dynamic, and your health needs may change over time. Be prepared to adapt your diet and lifestyle as needed. Listen to your body and make adjustments to stay aligned with your health goals.
- **Seeking Support:** Maintain a strong support network of friends, family, and health professionals. Their encouragement and advice

can help you navigate challenges and stay
motivated.

- **Setting New Goals:** Continuously set new health
  goals to keep yourself engaged and inspired.
  Whether it's trying new anti-inflammatory
  recipes, incorporating different physical
  activities, or focusing on mental well-being,
  having goals can provide direction and purpose.

Sharing Your Story and Inspiring Others

Sharing your story is a powerful way to inspire others
and contribute to a community of health and wellness.
Your experiences and insights can motivate others to
embark on their own health journeys. Here are some
ways to share your story:

- **Social Media and Blogging:** Use social media
  platforms or start a blog to share your journey,
  recipes, tips, and progress. Your story can reach a

wide audience and inspire others to make positive changes.

- **Community Involvement**: Get involved in local health and wellness communities. Participate in workshops, support groups, or volunteer opportunities to connect with others who share similar goals.

- **Personal Connections:** Share your experiences with friends, family, and colleagues. Personal stories can have a profound impact on those close to you and encourage them to prioritize their health.

- **Advocacy and Education:** Consider becoming an advocate for anti-inflammatory lifestyles. Educate others about the benefits of the diet and lifestyle changes, and support initiatives that promote health and wellness in your community.

Inspiring others not only reinforces your commitment to a healthy lifestyle but also creates a ripple effect that can lead to broader positive changes in society.

In conclusion, the journey ahead is about maintaining the positive changes you have made, continuing to learn and adapt, and sharing your story to inspire others. Reflecting on your progress helps you appreciate your achievements and stay motivated. By staying informed, seeking support, and setting new goals, you can sustain your health journey. Sharing your experiences can empower others to take control of their health and contribute to a community of wellness. Embrace this journey with enthusiasm and commitment, knowing that you have the power to lead a healthier, more vibrant life.

www.ingramcontent.com/pod-product-compliance
Lightning Source LLC
Chambersburg PA
CBHW070844250726
48662CB00003B/1355